Mediterranean Diet

Volume 1

By Anas Malla

Table of Contents

Introduction

I want to thank you and congratulate you for purchasing the book "**Mediterranean Diet Vol.1**"

Are you looking for a diet that is not a quick-fix but a long-term solution to get your body into shape and keep it that way? Are you tired of eating unhealthy foods and you believe that it is the right time to change your habits and start consuming healthy foods and nurture your body?

The people from the Mediterranean have a specific way of nutrition that has brought them incredible health benefits and increased longevity compared to the other parts of the world. The Mediterranean diet has been around for thousands of years, but it has only received the attention from nutritional experts during the last couple of decades.

The research undoubtedly confirmed – it's one of the best diets you can try to improve your health, get your body weight into order and improve your overall well-being. The nutritionists from around the world achieved consensus and agreed that the Mediterranean diet is the right way to go for everyone who is looking for a healthy way of nutrition.

The goal of this book is to get you familiar with all the information you need to know about the Mediterranean diet. It will be your number one guide and the only consultation you will need when starting your new regime of nutrition.

We will cover the following things:

- **Everything you need to know about the Mediterranean diet** – the first part of the book will give you an inside look into the history and the science behind the Mediterranean nutrition. Aside from that, you will find all about how the diet works and whether it fits into the busy and stressful life people are living today

- **Why you should try the Mediterranean diet** – once we cover the basics about your future way of nutrition, we will focus on the reasons why you should try and stick to the new regime of eating. You will find out why proper nutrition is crucial for your health, how Mediterranean diet can help you achieve your desired body weight, as well as read about numerous health benefits besides weight loss.

- **Why it is so healthy and delicious** – Mediterranean diet is based on the same healthy eating principles that nutritionists and health authorities from around the world recommend. You will get familiar with the Mediterranean food pyramid, which will explain in detail everything that you can eat when you make the switch to this nutrition, and you will find out why olive oil is so widespread in the Mediterranean countries. Aside from that, you will learn what you can drink during the diet, as well as how to find your way around when you are eating away from home or dining with your friends.

- **Living the Mediterranean style of life** – if you want long-term results from the Mediterranean diet, you will need to make some changes to your lifestyle, too. Fortunately, this book understands how hard it is to adjust your way of life and change your habits. That is why we are offering lifestyle tips and advice on how to avoid rookie mistakes when starting the Mediterranean diet.

The book tries to cover the Mediterranean diet from every possible angle, and I sincerely hope that it answers any question you might have when it comes to this regime of nutrition.

Thanks again for purchasing this book, I hope you enjoy it!

An Inside Look into the Mediterranean Diet

What Is Mediterranean Diet?

If you ever studied various cultures, you might already be familiar with a way of nutrition in the region of Mediterranean Sea, or more precisely in Greece, Italy, or Spain. Named after the area in which it was most used, this diet got the name Mediterranean.

When you say Mediterranean diet, the first thing that you should know is that there is no a single and utterly precise regime that can be called a Mediterranean diet. In fact, the way of nutrition differs from country to country. People have different eating habits in Malta than in Sardinia, and their diet varies depending on if their country of living is France or Greece.

We will talk more about the history of the Mediterranean diet later, but one thing that you have to know is that it changed over time thanks to the influence of various cultures around the Mediterranean region. During the last couple of decades, these countries also weren't immune to the emergence of fast food chains and junk food. However, for millennia before that, the actual Mediterranean diet became famous for its health benefits. The principles still apply, and they can still significantly contribute to your overall well-being, which is exactly why the term "Mediterranean" refers to the origin of this way of nutrition rather than particular foods.

The first professional that presented a concept of the Mediterranean diet was Dr. Walter Willet, a professor at the Harvard University. He said he based his suggestion of Mediterranean diet on the food patterns used in the south of Italy in the 1960s and the island Crete that belongs to Greece, which has the similar eating habits like the rest of that country.

The definition of the Mediterranean diet that Dr. Willet offered was:

"Everyone should eat a lot of plant-based foods. The desserts should consist of fresh fruits, and the primary source of fat should be olive oil. Yogurt, cheese, and other dairy products should also be used, while you can consume up to four eggs every week. You should restrict yourself from red meat, but you can consume poultry and fish in low to adequate amounts. Aside from eating in accordance with these rules, physical activity is also important for the Mediterranean diet."

The History behind the Mediterranean Diet

The Mediterranean diet, just like its name says, developed in Mediterranean countries. The Mediterranean region was a crossroad of different cultures and an essential link between the West and East for millenniums. The ports were used for developing both commerce and communication between countries that were diverse in cultures and eating habits. For these reasons, it doesn't come as a surprise that the Mediterranean diet and lifestyle were changed throughout history.

When we say Mediterranean diet, we mostly think of Greece and Italy as two countries that were the main participants in developing this way of nutrition. However, many foods used in the Mediterranean diet are foreign to their territories. Take, for example, various spices used. When pepper was brought from Asia, it was costly, but everyone loved adding it to their meals.

It also explains why many foods used in this way of nutrition is actually foreign to this territory. Egyptian had a significant influence on Greek and Roman culture, considering that they left the legacy of sourdough bread, which became essential for the Mediterranean diet. That is the reason why wheat became the foundation of the Greek and Roman way of nutrition in the ancient times.

Greek culture also appreciated nature, which explains the presence of olives in their way of nutrition. In fact, they considered the olive tree to be sacred, and they nurtured them with care. They also used wine during their celebrations, which completed the three basic items in the Mediterranean diet: olives, grapes, and wheat.

Once the Arabs came to the region with their cultural influence, they shaped the Mediterranean diet to value fruits and vegetables far more than up to that point. People in Iberian Peninsula (today's Portugal and Spain) adopted this principle and started adding a bunch of veggies and fruits to their eating habits. However, they also made sure to include a lot of fish. In fact, hunting was now much less present in this region, as well as raising cattle for the meat due to the land. That is why the people focused on fishing and including a lot of fatty fish in their way of nutrition.

The Fall of the Roman Empire

The Middle Ages brought us the final fall of the Roman Empire. The Germanic, who defeated Romans, did accept and take over some of the things from the Roman-Greek cuisine, such as bread and wine which became essential elements of the Christian culture. However, due to the influence of Celts, the Germanic people used meat as the totem of their nutrition, although they did discover that herbs can be important in adding the flavors and keeping the meat fresh.

A couple of centuries after that the Muslim conquests started and the Mediterranean region was an area of a big clash of different cultures. Muslims didn't eat pork and consume wine, both of which were associated with the Christian religion. Countries like Spain and Italy did maintain the lifestyle of eating ham products at this point.

When the Europeans started discovering the America ("the New World"), they brought back some foods that will remain in the Mediterranean diet up until today. The vegetables that you consume these days that came from America include tomato, potato, and eggplant, as well as cocoa or coffee.

The famine that occurred in Europe combined with vast destruction from wars caused that people were increasingly eating that food and it found its place in the culture of many civilizations in Europe. At the time, true Mediterranean nutrition was a poor man's diet. There was little meat because it wasn't available, and the main sources of foods were plants and legumes.

The Industrial Revolution led to the increase of the available food across the Mediterranean region. Women were included into the workforce, which meant that there was less time to prepare the food and cook. The population also increased, which lead to people discovering some crops that were incredibly productive, like spinach.

The last century saw the growth in consumption of the meat and dairy products and the decrease of cereals and bread. Furthermore, during the last 40-50 years, when you mention Italian or Greek cuisines, the first thing that comes to mind is lasagnas and pizzas followed by a long line of wine bottles. The truth is, however, that throughout the centuries, the concept of the true Mediterranean diet was far different.

It is an incredibly diverse way of nutrition that changed numerous times over the years. Asia, Africa, Europe, and America all had their influence in forming this way of lifestyle.

How Does It Work?

The most important thing to know is that a Mediterranean diet is not an exact plan of nutrition. Instead, it's a pattern that you can use to adjust your eating habits and make them healthier. Your body will be more than thankful if you do this, considering that Mediterranean diet has numerous health benefits.

Another excellent piece of news is that you should know is that it's not that hard to change your eating habits to Mediterranean. Of course, it always depends on the eating habits you had by now, but regardless of that, a strong will to change to a healthy lifestyle is what will take you to your goal.

The Basic Principles of the Mediterranean Diet

The Mediterranean diet sets on some basic principles that you should follow and incorporate into your eating habits. These are the most important rules of the true Mediterranean way of nutrition:

- **The vegetables are an absolute must** – plant-based foods make the core of the Mediterranean diet, and vegetables should be a part of your every meal. Aside from that, you also shouldn't be shy of other plant-based foods, such as fruits, legumes, and even cereals that are whole grain.

- **Restrict your consumption of meat** – if red meat is already out of your nutrition, that's great news because the Mediterranean diet almost entirely limits its use. Instead, you are welcome to consume poultry and fish in moderate amounts – they are an alternative that your body will more appreciate

- **Olive oil is the primary source of healthy fat** – olive oil is one of the key ingredients of the Mediterranean diet. You shouldn't be too shy when using it, considering that it has multiple health benefits and it's an excellent substitute for lard or butter.

- **Make sure to avoid processed foods** – you shouldn't avoid fat in the Mediterranean diet, but you should choose it carefully. That being said, you should avoid processed foods because there is a high chance that they contain a bunch of saturated fat that has proven to be extremely unhealthy for your heart and body.

- **Eat moderate amounts of dairy** – just like with fats, dairy is not forbidden during the Mediterranean diet, but you should choose it carefully. The acceptable options include various cheese, including goat and sheep versions, and low-fat milk.

- **You do not need extra salt** – if you are a person that likes salt, you should know that, in most cases, there is enough of it to eat in the food of the Mediterranean diet and you don't need to add any extra. If you have to adjust the flavoring a bit, you can use sea or Himalayan salt.
- **Nuts are an excellent way to go for a snack** – if you feel like having a snack you can always go for some nuts, as long as you decide for the unsalted ones. Alternatively, fresh fruits can be consumed as a fabulous snack substitute to biscuits or cakes.
- **Drink a lot of water** – water should be your go-to drink during the Mediterranean diet. Consume it whenever you are thirsty and feel free to drink as much as you like. Use it as a substitute for the sugary drinks you've been enjoying so far because they are an unhealthy option for you.

An Example of

a Mediterranean Day

As you can see from the principles, the Mediterranean diet is completely in line with the advice on healthy eating you've been getting from the experts on TV or even your parents. But, how does a Mediterranean nutrition plan for a day looks like?

Let's take a look at this example:

- **Breakfast** – go for a salad that includes red onion, chopped tomatoes, crumbled feta, some fresh herbs, and balsamic vinegar. Drizzle everything with olive oil and grab a slice of melon for the dessert. You can also enjoy a cup of Greek coffee.
- **Snack** – handful of nuts (hazelnuts, almonds, walnuts) or fresh fruit (a bunch or grapes, pear, figs)
- **Lunch** – vegetable mix prepared healthily on your stove or in your oven. A side dish can be a bowl of rice.
- **Second snack** – some walnuts or Greek yogurt with a bit of honey
- **Dinner** – grilled or baked fish with vegetable salad for a couple of times a week. On other evenings, enjoy salad from cooked greens with lemon juice and olive oil.
- **After-dinner dessert** – a small portion of fresh fruit (grapes, melons, figs)

What can we learn from this suggestion of nutrition? The first thing you notice is that you should have five or six meals every day. That is an important thing to remember because you need to eat regularly during the Mediterranean diet. Aside from making sure to have enough meals during the day, you should also plan on eating at proper time intervals in between. That means that you should pack three meals in three hours. Instead, try to divide them and have one every three to four hours.

All the other things that you noticed is that the foundations of the actual Mediterranean diet are completely in line with the suggested example. The vegetables are included in every meal; fruits are the chosen dessert, fish secures to get enough protein, while olive oil ensures the intake of monounsaturated fats you need.

Please note that you shouldn't use this example every day. I merely listed a suggestion on how a day might look like. Feel free to combine your meals any way you like as long as they are in line with the rules of the Mediterranean diet. Later in the book, we will discuss the Mediterranean food pyramid, which should give you a better idea of the portions of the food you can consume.

Is It for Busy People?

We know that life of today is full of events and stress and almost everybody is weak with time. The good news is that modern times come with some nifty devices, too, just like those instant pots, slow cookers, and other kitchen gadgets that help you prepare your food. All those make things like vegetable soups extremely simple to make. You can always make a meal that will last for a couple of days and keep it in the fridge until you want to eat it.

The majority of Mediterranean meals is suitable for preparing ahead, which makes the diet appropriate for busy people and those who are caught in the web of fast-paced life. However, you should always make sure to take your time to actually enjoy your meals and savor the delicious food you enjoy. That is of particular importance if you want to lose some weight with the Mediterranean diet because it will help you feel full sooner and not feel hunger for a longer time.

The Science behind the Mediterranean Diet

The Mediterranean diet isn't something that was created in a lab or by scientists. It is a lifestyle that existed and changed throughout more than 4,000 years. However, during the last century, the scientists became interested in the Mediterranean way of life. The reason was that they noticed a low death rate in Greece. That is why the American Rockefeller Foundation sponsored research to discover why that happens. It was unclear at the time, but to their surprise, they came to a conclusion that it might be because of the olive oil, which had a bunch of hidden health benefits.

The World Health Organization conducted an interesting project during the 1980s. The name of the project was Monica, and its goal was to keep full track of all the data of cardiovascular and coronary diseases around different parts of Europe. Among other things that they discovered, the most important data came from France. The diversity of the country enabled the South to be applying the Mediterranean diet, while the North included a lot of animal fats in their nutrition. The conclusion was obvious – people living in the South of France had significantly fewer cases of coronary and cardiovascular diseases than Strasbourg or Lille, cities that were located in the North.

At the beginning of the 21st century, 7000 participants from Spain agreed to take part in research that lasted for five years – from 2003 to 2007. The participants were divided into three groups – one that should follow a diet with at least 5 tablespoons a day of olive oil, the other group got the diet plan rich in nuts, while the third one was told to start a low-fat diet.

The results after five years showed the importance of fats – the group that was on the nutrition with olive oil had 30% fewer chances of experiencing a heart attack or a cardiovascular disease, while the ones on the nut diet were 28% less likely for that kind of an event than the people on a low-fat diet.

Antonia Trichopolou, a Greek scientist, conducted a study in 2003 in which she tried to quantify just how good the Mediterranean diet is. She observed a group of 22,000 Greeks for whom she assumed that were on a Mediterranean diet for a significant part of their lives. She made a scoring system and discovered that the closer the participants followed the diet, the lower was the mortality rate in their group.

It was this study that finally confirmed the health importance of the Mediterranean diet. Also, other studies proved the benefits of using the olive oil in your nutrition, but we will talk about that later in the book.

Why Is Mediterranean Diet Good for You?

The Importance of Proper Nutrition for Your Health

The everyday choices you make when it comes to food affect your health. It can influence how you feel today, as well as how you will feel tomorrow, and it will surely have a significant impact in the long-term.

The importance of proper nutrition for your health cannot be stressed enough. Poor choices when it comes to food can lead to numerous problems, which we can particularly notice in today's world of junk and other unhealthy foods.

Let me just give you a couple of statistical information. The research conducted in the United States in 2015 showed that 33% of the adults in the country have obesity issues. That means that every third adult in the U.S. is considered to be obese. Furthermore, 17% of kids and teenagers (the survey analyzed children and teens up to 19 years old) are obese.

Even if you don't have obesity issues, poor nutrition can bring you a host of health troubles. High blood pressure, increased the risk to develop a heart disease, type 2 diabetes, and even some cancer types are related to unhealthy eating habits. Numerous studies link poor nutrition with a bunch of adult chronic diseases, and the signs are too big to ignore, especially if you want to keep your health at a high level and decrease the risk of having trouble once you reach a mature age.

The good news is that it's never late to change your eating habits and start living a healthy lifestyle along with a healthy diet. Nutritionists around the world agree that Mediterranean diet is one of the best and the most efficient plans that you can stick to on a long-term basis.

Let's take a look at some of the vital advantages of this way of nutrition, starting with the issue that probably interests most of you – weight loss.

Weight Loss Benefits of the Mediterranean Diet

Many people decide to change their eating habits with one goal in their mind – lose extra pounds and get their body into shape. If you are among those people, you should know that you can lose weight with Mediterranean diet. However, one thing that you need to have in mind is that this diet is not a quick fix. Considering that it is a (complete) change of your way of eating, you should look at losing weight as only one of the primary goals that the Mediterranean nutrition brings.

There are diets out there that can help you lose pounds faster, but there is a good reason why you should try Mediterranean diet nonetheless. You see, it might take a bit more time to get to the desired weight, but once you achieve the goal, there is no chance that you will regain those extra pounds. On top of that, you will significantly improve your overall health, and you will eat some delicious food on your way to losing weight. Unlike the other weight-loss diets that come and go – the Mediterranean diet and its effects are there to stay. You can safely live with it on a long-term basis, and it has multiple benefits.

It's a pretty good deal – you get to eat foods full of flavor, make choices that will improve your health and contribute to you feeling better while losing pounds on the way. Let's take a look at few tips how controlling your portions and making smart food choices can help you get to the desired weight.

It's all about the Lifestyle

I'll repeat once again – Mediterranean nutrition is much more than a simple diet plan. That is why your focus should be on making lifestyle changes. Here are some quick tips that you can apply when it comes to changing your way of life:

- **Start with small changes** – it depends on how hard you consider transferring to the Mediterranean style of life is, but try implementing and noticing the small changes you managed to include into your daily routine.
- **Enjoy your meals** – take your time to sit down and eat each of your meals
- **Don't forget about physical activity** – taking a walk or exercising can play a major role in losing weight, which is why you should make sure to keep your physical activity at an adequate level

Calories, Calories, Calories

Losing weight has everything to do with calories, and that is the fact that any diet can't afford to miss. Let's just remember that calories are nothing but energy that your body needs for functioning and performing various activities during the day, starting from breathing up to cooking or exercising.

However, each one of us has a metabolic rate which decides how fast we burn those calories. Our metabolism depends on our gender, age, the level of fitness, and genetics.

The math with calories is rather simple – if you eat more calories than your body converts into energy during the day, there is no way that you can lose weight. If you want to get rid of those extra pounds, you need to eat fewer calories than you burn and make your body used the energy it stored throughout your body.

The important thing to emphasize is that the Mediterranean diet DOESN'T require you to keep track of your calories. To be more precise, there is no need to grab a calculator and calculate each calorie you eat. It's enough to control your portion sizes and exercise on a regular basis.

Lose Weight Even When Eating More

I have some good news for those of you who like to have considerable amounts of food on your plate. The Mediterranean diet approves eating a bunch of vegetables that are low in calories and discourages eating grains and meats, which are considered to have high calorie amounts. That means you can eat a lot of veggies and still lose weight.

The one thing to keep in mind is how much fat participates in your total daily amount of calories. The recommendable amount is around 35%, but one thing to make sure is to choose the healthy fats. Your primary source should be olive oil, but you can also eat fatty fish.

How to Control Your Food Cravings?

The good news is that the Mediterranean diet will actually help you suppress your appetite. If you make the right balance of fats and plant-based foods in your nutrition, you will achieve the feeling of satiety in the most natural way possible. The good way of making yourself feel full is to load up on fiber, so make sure to eat legumes, vegetables, and fruits in fiber.

Aside from that, you should make sure to avoid spikes in your blood sugar levels. They are most frequently the cause behind your food craving. Make sure that not more than 5 hours passes between two meals and that you don't skip any meals during the day. The Mediterranean diet suggests that you should grab something to eat every three to five hours. Good advice I can give is to eat as soon as you feel hungry. That way you will eat less until you feel full. Aside from that, eating foods that are rich in protein but low in fats can slow down the digestion of the food in your body. Fish, nuts, and beans can all contribute to you feeling full for a longer period of time.

Finally, you should know that stress can also be the reason why you have food cravings. That is why you should find some time during the day to relax. A meditation and other deep breathing techniques can contribute to feeling less stressed. Aside from that, make sure that you get enough sleep, drink enough water, and exercise, which can also help to manage your stress hormones.

Health Benefits beyond Losing Weight

Mediterranean diet has a bunch of amazing health benefits that can contribute to the overall state of your organism. Let's take a look at some of them:

Improves the Health of Your Heart

Some of the foods consumed in the Mediterranean diet are rich in omega-3 acids and monounsaturated fats, which are proven to be helpful in decreasing the risk of heart disease. The olive oil also contains ALA (alpha-linoleic acid), which can reduce the possibility of death from cardiac issues for up to 30 percent and the risk of a sudden heart attack by up to 45 percent.

Another positive effect of using the olive oil in your nutrition is related to blood pressure. Studies conducted by Warwick Medical School proved that those who consume olive oil of the highest quality had decreased blood pressure compared to those using sunflower and other refined oils. The reason why olive oil manages to lower hypertension is thanks to the fact that it releases nitric oxide in your body, which helps to keep your arteries clear and dilated.

Helps Prevent and Treat Diabetes

The Mediterranean diet is rich in anti-inflammatory foods, which means that it helps with the diseases that are connected to chronic inflammation. Type 2 diabetes is among them.

The reason why the Mediterranean diet helps prevent diabetes and keep your blood sugar levels in order is that it puts excess insulin under control. Also, the Mediterranean style of eating means that you are consuming foods that are low in sugar and what better way there is to keep your blood sugar levels under control than that one?

The only sugar that you eat in the Mediterranean diet comes from fruit. Add to that the fact that you don't consume a bunch of foods rich in carbs and the fact that you should keep your physical activity at an adequate level and you secure that your blood sugar levels are stable.

Helps Prevent Cancer

The European Journal of Cancer Prevention published an article in 2012 that shows the high amounts of antioxidants, fiber, and polyphenols present in vegetables, fruits, and olive oil, as well as a balanced ratio of fatty acids omega-3 and omega-6, all contribute to helping in the prevention of cancer.

The antioxidants can stop cell mutation, protect your DNA from damage, as well as delay tumor growth and lower inflammation. Some studies suggest that the olive oil also helps in preventing cancer, and notably decreases the risk of bowel and colon cancers.

Reduces the Risk of Alzheimer Disease

Cognitive disorders are something that occurs a lot more often than you might think. As the years go by, dementia and memory loss can happen to all of us. The reason why that occurs is that dopamine, a chemical crucial for thought processing, can't reach our brain in sufficient levels.

Anti-inflammatory fruits and vegetables combined with healthy fats from nuts and olive oil are the winning combinations to fight cognitive decline that is age-related. The Mediterranean diet is one of the natural ways to treat Alzheimer's, as well as a treatment for Parkinson's disease.

It Affects Your Mood in a Good Way

The Mediterranean diet can also affect your mood and help you relax and de-stress. Although this is done indirectly and not through the things you eat, it's an effect that we cannot neglect. The Mediterranean lifestyle suggests that you should have adequate physical activity. Exercising is an excellent way to reduce stress and get more relaxed.

Aside from that, an important thing to do when being on a Mediterranean diet is to make time for meals. If you are living with your partner or your family, that can give you some time to spend together during lunch or dinners, which in turn helps you bond with your close one and makes you feel better.

The Most Important Benefit of All

The most important reason why the Mediterranean diet is ideal for you lies in the fact that it is a long-term way of nutrition. Numerous other diets are not healthy over long periods of time, but with Mediterranean way of nutrition – the longer you stick to the new eating habits, the bigger the benefits. It's the nutrition that you can use for the rest of your lifetime and maximize its benefits.

Risks and Concerns

There aren't many risks and concerns related to the Mediterranean diet because it follows the nutrition tips that even the official health authorities offer. However, there are several things to keep into account:

Keep track of your calcium levels

Dairy is the largest source of calcium in most diets around the world. However, the Mediterranean diet suggests that you should restrict your dairy to moderate amounts, and consume just some of the products, such as low-fat yogurt, cheese, and low-fat milk. Your choices are to include vegetables rich in calcium into your diet (kale, broccoli, spinach, soy beans) or make sure that you consume enough cheese and yogurt. Alternatively, you can add skim milk to your way of nutrition.

It shouldn't be too hard to secure enough calcium for your organism, but it can't hurt to be careful and keep track of its levels.

Watch the Amount of Fats

Aside from carefully choosing the healthy fats, another thing to make sure is that you don't go (too much and often) over the border of the suggested fat levels in your nutrition. The total daily fat consumption should be around 35%, and you should make sure not to exceed the recommended amount. Be especially careful if and when consuming saturated fats.

You Will Have to Learn to Cook

The truth is – the Mediterranean diet relies on your abilities in the kitchen. There are enough simple recipes available, but if you have never entered your kitchen before, now would be the right time. Once you get a grip on everything, you won't have any trouble even preparing the recipes that require advanced cooking skills. Who knows, you might discover that chef trapped deep within you!

What Makes Mediterranean Diet Healthy & Delicious?

Mediterranean diet lies on various principles of healthy eating that people applied for centuries. The important thing to know when starting with your new way of nutrition is what foods to eat and what to avoid. That is what we will cover in this section along with the Mediterranean food pyramid, which should help you get an inside look at all the available foods on this diet.

The Secret of Olive Oil

In the first part of the book, we discussed the science behind the Mediterranean diet and the fact that it can lower mortality rate and improve your cardiovascular health. Although the Mediterranean way of nutrition is rich with different healthy food, there is one item that deserves to get an entire subsection. Say hello to its majesty – olive oil.

It is this oil that was marked as the crucial ingredients that should be a major component of every Mediterranean diet. When the researchers compared the way of nutrition in Greece and Southern European countries to the eating habits in other countries, they concluded that it was the olive oil and olives that the Greeks had to thank for their extended lifespan and fewer cases of cardiovascular issues.

Olives are packed with antioxidants and polyphenols, and they are a fantastic source of monounsaturated fats. They have numerous benefits on your overall health, with the emphasis on heart health.

The important thing to know is how to choose the perfect olive oil for you. As you can assume, not all olive oil are created equal. That is why it is important to make a good choice when it comes to the product you buy. The highest grade an olive oil can have is that it is "extra virgin." It means that it's made mechanically and no excessive heat or chemicals were used in the production process. Loosely translated, it's the best olive oil you can buy for the money.

Another thing to make sure is that there is a harvesting or expiration date on the label of your olive oil. You see, the more recent the date when olives were harvested, the better the oil. Choose the one with the most recent harvesting date to ensure that it has maximum health benefits for you.

So, just how much olive oil should you use per day? The studies show that Greeks consume on average 5-6 tablespoons of olive oil per day. You can use it in any way you want – to prepare your food in a cooker or drizzle over your favorite salad.

Mediterranean Food Pyramid

There is an excellent concept that you can follow when it comes to choosing your food on the Mediterranean diet, and it's called the food pyramid. It is completely adjusted to the modern way of life after a consensus was achieved by the nutritional, agriculture, and sociology experts, as well as relevant international entities.

The food pyramid functions like this – the base level contains the food that you should most often include in your Mediterranean diet. The following levels on top of the ground one include food that you should consume far less often. We will now consider the pyramid from the ground up to see which foods you can include in your Mediterranean eating habits.

The Ground Level

Non-Starchy Vegetables

Vegetables are the foundation of most of your meals in the Mediterranean diet. However, you should pay attention when choosing your vegetables, and non-starchy options should be your primary choice. These include broccoli, artichokes, cabbage, carrots, celery, tomatoes, onion, cucumber, eggplant, zucchini, green beans, salad greens, peppers, mushrooms, beets, Brussels sprouts, cucumber, and cauliflower.

Your aim should be to consume 4-8 servings of non-starchy vegetables every day. A cup of raw vegetables or ½ cup of their cooked alternatives is considered as a single serving.

Starchy Vegetables and Whole Grains

Starchy vegetables are the other type of veggies at your disposal. They include corn, peas, and potatoes. They should also find their way into your meals, but in somewhat less amount than their non-starchy counterparts. In fact, they are in the same group with the whole grains because they achieve the same effect of ensuring you are in control of your hunger through keeping your stomach full for a longer period of time.

If you were wondering why you should choose whole grains over the processed versions, the answer is simple. They will mess with your triglyceride and blood sugar levels far less, which makes them more appropriate for the Mediterranean diet. On top of that, they are high in fiber, which secures the energy your body needs to function each day.

You should aim to have 4-6 servings of starchy vegetables and whole grains during the day. A serving is considered to be a piece of whole wheat bread or a small (6-inch) pita. You can also go for ½ cup cooked brown rice or whole wheat pasta. The choices of whole grain cereal include ½ cup cooked quinoa, cracked wheat, or oatmeal. As for the veggies, one serving is considered to be ½ cup of corn, potatoes, or peas.

Fruit

Fruit is also located at the ground level of the Mediterranean food pyramid, which makes it imperative to consume when on this way of nutrition. There are no bad choices when it comes to fruits, but make sure to always go with fresh fruit whenever you can. Be careful with choosing frozen fruits and make sure to read the label of the product because versions with no sugar added are only acceptable.

Canned and dried fruits should also be avoided whenever possible because of the sugar, as well as the fruit juices you can buy on the store shelves – they are, in most cases, full of artificial ingredients. On the other hand, you can drink natural fresh juice you squeezed yourself, but whole fruit is a better option because it will secure higher amounts of fiber.

The amount of fruits you should consume each day is between 2 and 4 servings. One fresh fruit is considered as a single serving, as well as a ½ cup of fruit juice. You can use them for snacks and desserts, and they are excellent substitutes for options rich in (usually unhealthy) fats.

Nuts and Legumes

Nuts may have a bit more calories than what you would like if you are on a weight-loss regime of nutrition, but each bite brings a lot of nutrients into your body. Nuts are rich in healthy unsaturated fats, which are able to increase good cholesterol levels without adjusting the bad cholesterol, too. Aside from that, they are rich in fiber and protein, which is something that also goes for legumes. In fact, legumes can be your primary source of protein when you eat meatless meals.

You should have 1-3 servings of nuts and legumes per day. When it comes to nuts, a serving is about 20 peanuts, 8 pecans or walnuts, 14 almonds, 1 tablespoon of peanut butter or 2 tablespoons of sesame and sunflower seeds. As for legumes, enjoy a ½ cup of cooked beans (black, kidney, soy, garbanzo, navy), as well as lentils or split peas.

Herbs and Spices

The biggest complaint people have when they start a new diet is that their food lacks in flavor. Fortunately, the Mediterranean healthy eating habits will secure that you enjoy flavorful foods while you consume the right food for your organism. Instead of adding much salt and risking your blood pressure to rise, you can try herbs and spices, such as parsley, oregano, dill, basil, sage, and mint. They are healthier and packed with antioxidants.

Feel free to add herbs and spices to your food whenever you like.

Physical Activity

It doesn't fit into food, but it is at the ground level for a good reason. If you want to maintain good health, it is essential to have regular physical activity. Everything that comes to your mind falls into this category, starting from doing yard work or helping your neighbor move, up to daily running, swimming, or working out in the gym.

Another thing located at the bottom of the pyramid is enjoying meals. It's crucial to make enough time and sit down to eat your breakfast, lunch, or dinner, whether you are doing it alone or with someone.

Level One: Fish and Seafood

Fish is a vital source of protein for your nutrition, but it is particularly valuable thanks to Omega-3 fatty acids, which positively affect your heart and brain health. The same goes for shellfish and other seafood, which you can freely enjoy 2 to 3 times every week.

You should go for fish that fall into the fatty categories, such as herring, salmon, mackerel, or sardines. Feel free to sauté, grill, broil, roast, bake or poach your fish while preparing it. One serving of fish is about three ounces of it.

Poultry

Poultry is another adequate source of protein, which is why it should find its place in your Mediterranean diet for once to three times a week. However, there are some tricks to apply to avoid saturated fat, which is not good news for you. Make sure to remove the skin from the chicken when you eat it and always stick to the white meat.

One serving of poultry is about three ounces of it.

Level Two: Dairy

When it comes to dairy, it's a rather tricky turf. For example, egg yolks can cause you some trouble with bad cholesterol, which is why you should consider restricting from consuming whole eggs if you already have high cholesterol. That being said, you can feel free to eat egg whites as much as you like.

When it comes to other dairy products, high-quality cheeses can be consumed several times a week (feta, goat, or soy cheese). When it comes to milk and yogurt, you should always go for the non-fat or low-fat (1%) versions.

The problem with dairy is that you should restrict the portions to between one and three servings per day, but you also need to make sure to get enough calcium. The good idea is to add skim milk to your nutrition or drink soy yogurt and soy milk which are calcium-fortified. If you are not a fan of any of this, you can consider adding a nutritional supplement that contains vitamin D and calcium.

Make sure to keep track of your levels of calcium when you start the Mediterranean diet to find out if you need supplements. A serving of dairy is considered to be a cup of non-fat milk or yogurt or an ounce of low-fat cheese.

Top of the Pyramid: Sweets

Top of the pyramid contains food that you should practically avoid at all costs. That being said, you are allowed to make an occasional slip up (like, once a month), but if you want to live the true Mediterranean lifestyle, you shouldn't eat any of the food listed here.

Sweets are the first thing on the top of the Mediterranean food pyramid. They usually have a high amount of sugar, and they are processed, which means they are also rich in saturated fats, which affect your heart health and overall well-being in a bad way. Aside from that, sweets don't have any nutritional value (or their value is meager). That is what puts them in the category of the food that is best left out from the plan of nutrition.

The bad news is that there are a bunch of sweets at your disposal as soon as you enter the store. However, avoid those chocolates (if you have to, dark chocolate can be an adequate dessert), cakes, biscuits, and even fruit juices, to which artificial sweeteners and other ingredients are added only to extend their shelf life.

If you are looking for a dessert, find a fruit that you like instead. They have higher nutritional value but are lower in calories.

Red Meat

Although the western culture nurtures eating red meat that is an entirely wrong move which severely affects your overall health, especially in long-term. Red meat has incredibly high portions of saturated fat, which is why you should limit their use to a couple of times per month (not more than three or four).

When you do go for red meat, always choose beef, veal, or lamb, and make sure to select lean cuts. That way, you will avoid most of those saturated fats that are essentially bad for you.

What to Drink during Mediterranean Diet?

Aside from the dilemmas on what you can eat and how much, another important part of the Mediterranean diet concerns what you should drink. Let's take a look at beverages that are allowed for this way of nutrition:

Water

Similar to many other (healthy) diets, water is an essential item in your diet. Authentic Mediterranean diet also emphasizes the importance of water and recommends that you should drink at least six glasses of water every day.

What makes water so great? First of all, it doesn't contain any calories, which means there is no effect on your body weight. Aside from that, water is a major component of our bodies. In case you didn't know, about 60% of our organisms is made from water. That is why we have to ensure that our water intake is adequate because, that way, we will ensure that our bodily functions work properly. It's something you've undoubtedly experienced in your life – when you are thirsty, you start noticing that you are feeling a bit lack of energy. Dehydration can cause serious health issues, which is why we need to drink enough water.

You can start from six glasses of water every day. However, one thing to keep in mind is that each human body is different and the amount of water that your organism demands may vary from mine or someone else's. Aside from genetics, water requirements also depend on physical activity, the environment you are in, and your body composition and mass.

That is why you should treat six glasses only as a starting point. Of course, this recommendation assumes that you will get a portion of your daily requirements through other drinks and even foods you consume. So that you know, it's completely in line with the Mediterranean style of life to drink water during the meal.

Coffee and Tea

Ever since the coffee was brought to the Mediterranean region, people over there drank it after breakfast or any other meal. However, there is an important thing you should know. Coffee doesn't mean that you can drink those large lattes that have almost a gallon of milk and who are topped with whipped cream. That type of coffee should be avoided at all cost.

On the other hand, you can freely drink regular coffee during the Mediterranean diet. However, too much coffee is also not the healthiest option for you, which is why you should restrict yourself to having no more than three cups per day.

Tea has been recently included in the Mediterranean diet, although the people from the region don't exactly have the habit of drinking it. However, most teas have antioxidants and polyphenols, which can help our health. For those of you who are on the weight-loss regime, you should also consider drinking green tea.

Milk and Yogurt

We already covered this within the section of dairy, but let's analyze everything once again. Milk should not be the main drink of the Mediterranean diet regardless of its type. However, you can occasionally allow yourself a glass of low-fat or skim milk. You can also try almond milk, which has the base in nuts, which means that it is rich in unsaturated fats that can improve your heart health.

As for yogurt, Greek yogurt should be your choice. Just like with milk, keep the amounts of it moderate. The important thing to know is that you should avoid fruit yogurts you can buy in supermarkets because it usually has added sugar.

Fruit Juices

Fruit juices can be an alternative when you don't feel like having a whole fruit. However, you should know that squeezed fruit juices have fewer nutrients and fiber than its whole counterparts. If you are looking for great options, try grape or berry juice, which can improve your heart health.

Another thing to remember is that you should avoid artificial fruit juices you can buy in supermarkets. They have all kinds of artificial ingredients, especially added sugar that will cause blood sugar spikes and can lead to increased hunger and obesity issues.

Wine

Although the general recommendation is not to drink alcohol, the Mediterranean diet will tolerate a glass of red wine now and then. According to some studies, it can help in adjusting your good and bad cholesterol levels, making it healthy for the heart. However, you should know that consuming alcohol can have severe consequences and can cause great health and social problems.

Eating Out Guide

The hardest time to resist temptation when it comes to food is when you are eating out with your friends. However, the Mediterranean lifestyle emphasizes the importance of social life, and we don't want you losing your contacts just because you are trying to lose some weight or eat healthier.

Fortunately, there are some bullet-proof tips that you can use when you are eating out. Take a look at them:

Appetizers – you probably can relate to this situation – you sit down at a nice restaurant, and the waiter brings butter and bread along with the appetizers. It's hard to resist this temptation, which is why the best idea is to ask whoever is serving to skip that part and not bring you butter or bread onto the table. Another thing you should make sure is that you don't eat anything fried for an appetizer. On the other hand, you can choose some vegetable salads, grilled vegetables and even steamed or raw fish, as well as soups that are based on vegetable broth. Another good idea is to ask your friends to share a single portion of appetizer to make sure you can control your portion.

Main courses – the first tip you need to apply is to avoid fried food at all costs. Other than that, you should use the same guidelines you use at home. Vegetable-based dishes are always an excellent choice, but fish or poultry (skinless) also can be considered. If you think that you can give yourself a free pass, you can choose a lean cut of beef like filet mignon (don't do that unless you really feel like eating the meat).

One thing you need to take into consideration is the sauces that accompany the dish. There shouldn't be any butter, cream, or sunflower oil in the sauce (olive oil is acceptable). Ask the waiter to give you information about the sauce and, if it doesn't fit with your diet, ask for a different sauce or just ask him to bring it on the side for your friends. You can also ask the waiter if the restaurant can substitute the ingredients that don't fit into your way of nutrition. In most cases, they will be glad to comply and fulfill your request. In that case, don't forget to be generous when tipping the waiter.

Unfortunately, the portions that restaurants serve these days are usually generous (although it might seem different). That is why you should try not to finish the entire plate. Ask the waiter to pack a half of the main course for you to bring home.

During eating, make sure to savor every bite and enjoy the meal (remember how we talked about that being important?). Also, as soon as you feel like you are not hungry anymore, ask the waiter to take your plate away.

Other guidelines

Just like it would be a home, fruit is your best option for a dessert in the restaurant. Alternatively, you can go with a cup of coffee or herbal tea. While we are on the topic of drinks, let's mention that water should be your go-to drink (if you are allowed, you can drink a glass of wine, but you need a strong will to keep it at that).

Living the Mediterranean Style of Life

I'm sure you have found yourself saying in the evening on more than one occasion:

"Tomorrow, I'm turning a new leaf and starting a fresh way of life!"

The next thing you know is that you get up in the morning and continue with the old habits. Changing your lifestyle is hard, and that is what you will need to do if you want to make a successful switch to a Mediterranean diet. Yes, nutrition might play the important part of any diet, but that's not the only change you are going to feel. This section of the book will focus on the tips that will make your transition to the new lifestyle easier, as well as on the mistakes that you need to avoid.

Lifestyle Tips for Mediterranean Diet

Think About What You Want to Achieve

Why are you starting the Mediterranean diet? Do you want to lose those extra pounds or you want to make a complete change and start living a healthier life and nurture your body? Regardless of what your goal is, make sure to set it on the first day of the Mediterranean diet. It might be a good idea to write it down and remind yourself of it whenever you feel like you are tempted by wrong foods.

Feel free to be vivid in describing what you want to achieve – write down how you imagine that you will look like after some time on the Mediterranean diet. Take note about how you want to feel (full of energy, stronger than today…), too. However, make sure that you've set realistic objectives and that you placed them in an achievable timeframe. You don't want to make goals that are too hard to achieve and bum yourself out.

Remind Yourself That It Is Going Well

Did you just endure your first week on the new regime of nutrition? Have you noticed a small decrease in the number of pounds you have? Do you look better to yourself when you stand in front of a mirror?

Well, I think that it's the right time to congratulate yourself for those results! Yes, you are still on your way to the ultimate goal you've set, but you need to make sure to recognize the little achievements you made in between. If you notice the small steps you are making to a big goal, it will give you a boost of confidence and motivation to continue and the following days of the diet will be easier.

Try to Focus on the Things You Can Eat

Mediterranean diet is not all that restricting. Yes, it is strict when it comes to giving up junk and sugary foods, but only because that is the right thing to do. That is why the best thing to do is not to think of all the things you can't eat but focus on those that you can.

I'm positive that you can find a lot of stuff that you like that will fit into your Mediterranean diet. If you feel like the transition is tough, try to implement the changes gradually. Don't forget, any diet you try shouldn't be overbearing or too hard, especially for your mind. If needed, give yourself a couple of months to adjust to a new way of nutrition and allow yourself an occasional slip-up here and there. Just remember – the stronger you adhere to the rules of the Mediterranean diet, the better and faster results it will provide.

Prepare Your Meals in Advance

More importantly, have a plan for at least several meals ahead. Get the ingredients you need and prepare the food for tomorrow in the evening. That way you will avoid the race with time and the stress of being late for work or missing a meal.

Another thing that you will achieve by planning is to keep track of the amount of calories and fat you are consuming. If you know you are going out with friends tonight and you might have fish or poultry, it might be a good idea to have a simple lunch filled with non-starchy vegetables.

Explore the Recipes and Eat Different Stuff

According to numerous studies, one of the main reasons people were giving up on their diet after several days is because they were bored with it. They were fed up of eating the same food for days, and it didn't give them any feeling of satisfaction whatsoever.

Fortunately for you, there are literally thousands of recipes available out there that fit into the Mediterranean diet. The only thing that you should do is explore and find the ones that suit you or that you feel like eating right now. You don't have to eat steamed vegetables every day. It' s always a nice idea to play with different spices and herbs that can significantly improve the flavor of your food and give you the feeling like you are eating something new every time.

Hit the Local Markets

Don't restrict yourself to the nearest supermarket or store to your home. Instead, hit the local markets and check out what kind of different vegetables and fruits you can find over there. Whole foods are the key to the Mediterranean diet, and I'm sure you can find a bunch of them at the local market and make your trip worthwhile.

Make Some Time for Yourself during the Day

We are living in stressful times, but regardless of how busy you are during the day, you should always make sure to make some time for yourself, even if it's only ten minutes or half an hour. During that leisure time, do whatever relaxes you – meditate, watch a movie or enjoy your favorite hobby, such as painting. Relaxation time is the best way to relieve yourself of the stress you have accumulated during the day.

Don't Compare Yourself to Others

That is just common sense and doesn't have anything to do with the fact that you are on a diet or not. It is especially important if you are on a new way of nutrition with the goal of losing weight. You see, each human body is unique and works at its own pace. So, if you've started the diet the same day as your friend and he/she has better results after several weeks, that's not a reason to worry.

I'm sure that you are also making progress. Focus on that and make sure to adhere to the diet guidelines even more than before. Have the goal you want to reach in mind and make sure that is the only thing you are focusing on.

Rookie Mistakes to Avoid

Don't Let Your Kitchen Be Empty

The easiest way to slip up when adhering to a diet is not to have anything to eat when you start feeling the hunger. That is why your kitchen should be filled with vegetables that you can whip up into a salad in a matter of minutes. You should also store some fruit so that you can grab a snack whenever you feel like it.

The studies show that if you need to prepare a meal once you feel the hunger, it's incredibly easy to give in to temptation and order some junk food or grab that bag of chips that's been in your cupboard for months.

Don't Skip Your Meals

We already covered the importance of eating your meals on a regular basis. Skipping them can lead to blood sugar spikes, which means that the diet might have less effect than desired. There should be a timeframe of three to five hours between every meal, and you should make sure to have five or six of them per day. One thing that can help you in making sure not to skip your meals is the first advice in this subsection – always make sure to have something to snack on in your kitchen.

You Are Not Getting Enough Sleep

Not getting an adequate amount of sleep can increase your appetite and instigate food cravings. Aside from that, it can make you feel moody and therefore increase your stress levels. The experts say that getting six to eight hours of good night sleep is essential and can substantially contribute to the overall state of your organism.

You Are Not Drinking Enough Water

It's important to stay hydrated during the Mediterranean diet. Aside from the fact that it helps your bodily functions to work correctly, it assists in releasing the toxins trapped inside your organism. On top of that, it's not a rare occurrence that people mistake hunger for thirst. So, the next time you are feeling hungry, take a glass of water and wait for 10 minutes – you might find out that you were not hungry after all.

You Stray Off-Course Because of One Mistake

Let me tell you one harsh truth – when you start a new regime of nutrition, it's bound that you will make some mistakes. If you are used to eating sweets, sooner or later, you won't be able to resist, and you will indulge your sweet tooth by eating a piece of cake or something like that.

When that happens, the important thing to know is that it is not the end of the world. You shouldn't be bummed because you made a single mistake. However, you should make sure that you get back on the right track starting with the following meal. Act as if nothing happened and you've had a fruit instead of that unhealthy snack and continue with your Mediterranean diet just like you did up to that point.

Of course, try to ensure to make mistakes as rarely as possible in order to maximize the results of the diet.

Conclusion

Thank you again for purchasing this book!

I hope this book was able to help you understand the **Mediterranean diet** and all its benefits correctly.

As you could notice, the primary focus of the Mediterranean diet is to bring you long-term benefits and improve your overall health. It achieves this through its principles of what you should and what you shouldn't eat, as well as on focusing on regular physical activity. You will get all the nutrients you need from plant-based foods, which make the ideal combination with an occasional portion of fish or poultry.

It's not easy to make a change to your lifestyle, but it's important to know that staying strong will secure that you will reap maximum benefits from the Mediterranean diet. If you were not a fan of vegetables and fruit before, it might be harder to make the transition to the plant-based diet, but remember – the improvement of your health and the fact that you will get your body in shape are worth it.

Finally, if you enjoyed this book, then I'd like to ask you for a favor, would you be kind enough to leave a review for this book on Amazon? It'd be greatly appreciated.

Visit the link below to leave a review:
https://www.amazon.com/review/create-review

For more information, please check out my blog at:
Mastering-life.com

Thank you and good luck!

Preview of
"Ketogenic Diet" Book

Introduction

I want to thank you and congratulate you for downloading the book **"Ketogenic Diet"**

This book contains proven steps and strategies on how to lose weight with the ketogenic diet.

I used to have a big problem with obesity. I was constantly eating and overeating unhealthy and junk food and I didn't lift a finger when it comes to activity. One day I've decided – things have got to change!

The ketogenic diet helped me not only achieve my ideal weight (I lost over 50 pounds), but it also improved my body composition by getting rid of that stored fat in my belly and other areas.

Now, I look and feel much better! I have so much energy and I can go on and on without feeling tired. That is why I've decided to share with you the secret of achieving the perfect state of your organism with the help of the ketogenic diet.

Here's what we will cover in this book:

- What is ketogenic diet, how it works and why it is a perfectly healthy way to lose weight

- How to calculate the number of macronutrients you need?

- What food should you eat and avoid during keto?

- 4-week ketogenic diet plan as a suggestion

- More than 30 completely keto-friendly recipes!

And much more!

I've used my own experience of going through keto to help explain it to you in the best way. I noted down all the questions I had and tried to answer them for you in this book.

Everything you need to know about the ketogenic diet is in one place – here.

Thanks again for downloading this book, I hope you enjoy it!

Chapter 1 – Ketosis Explained

Ketosis is a regular metabolic process in our body and it happens on an everyday basis. It is a metabolic state where your body uses ketone bodies in the blood for some of its energy supply.

The human body is extremely adjustable and it can process different nutrients into the fuel it needs to work. Carbs, fats, and proteins are all potential sources of energy supply. When you eat a lot of carbohydrates or proteins, your body breaks them down into glucose (also known as blood sugar). Glucose is then used in creating an energy molecule called ATP, which your organism uses for maintenance and daily activities within the body.

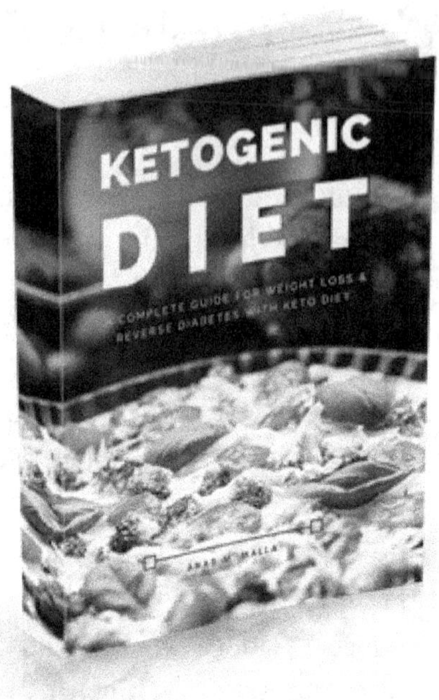

Believe it or not, our body uses most of the nutrients we intake just for daily maintenance. However, if you eat enough food, the chances are that there will be an excessive amount of glucose which the body doesn't require at the moment. In that case, one of the two things happens:

- **Glycogenesis** – the excess amount of glucose is converted to glycogen and stored in your muscles and liver

- **Lipogenesis** – once your body believes that there is enough glycogen in your liver and muscles, the remaining glucose will be converted into fats and stored within your body

Ketosis is a process that happens when your organism is out of glycogen or glucose. In cases when your body can't access food, it will start burning fat and creating ketones (energy molecules). This process usually occurs when you are sleeping, so it is a completely normal metabolic state of the organism. The human body has a natural ability to switch metabolic pathways.

When your body starts burning fat and making fatty acids, the end result of the process is the creation of ketones. These molecules are then used by your brain and muscles as a fuel. In most cases, the human body uses glucose as the main source of its energy supply. However, once the carbohydrate or protein intake is low, your body will simply use fatty acids as a natural alternative.

What Is Ketosis and How Does It Work?

Ketosis is a process that occurs when your body is out of glycogen or glucose and it starts using consumed and stored fat as a fuel for maintenance and daily activities. It is a metabolic state your body should be in when you are on a ketogenic diet.

The study conducted by the University of California shows that the human organism actually prefers using ketones. In fact, it is about 70% more efficient than when running on glucose. If you think about it from an evolutionary point of view, it makes perfect sense. Our ancestors didn't have constant access to glucose. Hell, they didn't even have regular access to food.

Instead, their body was using the fat from the animal they ate.

The Process Explained

Your liver breaks down the consumed or stored fat and releases fatty acid molecules and glycerol. The next step is breaking down the fatty acids further. This process is called ketogenesis and it produces a ketone body by the name of acetoacetate.

Your body converts acetoacetate into one of the two types of ketones:

- **BHB (beta-hydroxybutyrate)** – after your body gets adapted to the state of ketosis, your muscles will use the acetoacetate to convert it to BHB and your body will then use it as brain fuel

- **Acetone** – lesser amounts of acetone are converted into glucose, but most of it is thrown out as waste. This might lead to a characteristic breath smell that ketogenic dieters are familiar with

As your organism gets used to ketosis, your body will expel a lesser amount of ketones. This doesn't mean that the process is slowing down. It just means that your body got better at feeding the brain with BHB as an energy supply.

You do need glucose in small amounts to maintain good health, which is why your organism creates it with acetone. The liver is there to make sure that you have enough glucose in your blood.

Unlike glucose, there is absolutely no need for carbohydrates. More than 50% of the excessive amount of proteins is turned into glucose. That is why eating carbs is a bad thing if you are on a ketogenic diet – it can knock you out of the state of ketosis.

Ketosis vs. Starvation

The state of ketosis is not the same as fasting. Starvation occurs when you don't have any food source whatsoever. It leads to your body using your muscle tissues to make the glucose it needs.

On the other hand, ketosis is a healthy way to lose additional pounds. The ketogenic process helps your body use the amount of fat it has stored and helps you preserve your muscle tissue.

Go to this link to check out the rest of the

"Ketogenic Diet":

http://amzn.to/2ps3ePm

Check Out My Other Books

Below you'll find some of my other popular books that are popular on Amazon and Kindle as well. Simply click on the links below to check them out.

Alternatively, you can visit my "Author Page" on Amazon to see other work done by me:

Anas Malla: http://amzn.to/2nzCevB

- **Alkaline Diet V.1**
http://amzn.to/2shityl

- **Ketogenic Diet**
http://amzn.to/2ps3ePm

- **Ketogenic Bread Cookbook V.1**
http://amzn.to/2m8hixm

- **Ketogenic Bread Cookbook V.2**
http://amzn.to/2r3qsPJ

- **Ketogenic Bread Cookbook V.3**
http://amzn.to/2r3Af8j

- **Instant Pot Ketogenic Cookbook V.1**
http://amzn.to/2o4oCfP

- **Instant Pot Ketogenic Cookbook V.2**
http://amzn.to/2o4oCfP

- **Ketogenic Fat Bombs V.1**
http://amzn.to/2qDgS4U

- **Minimalist Living**
http://amzn.to/2phTu8M

- **Conversation Tactics**
http://amzn.to/2oj23Qg

If the links do not work, for whatever reason, you can simply search for these titles on the Amazon website to find them.

9 781987 722390